THE ULTIMATE DASH DIET COOKBOOK FOR SENIORS

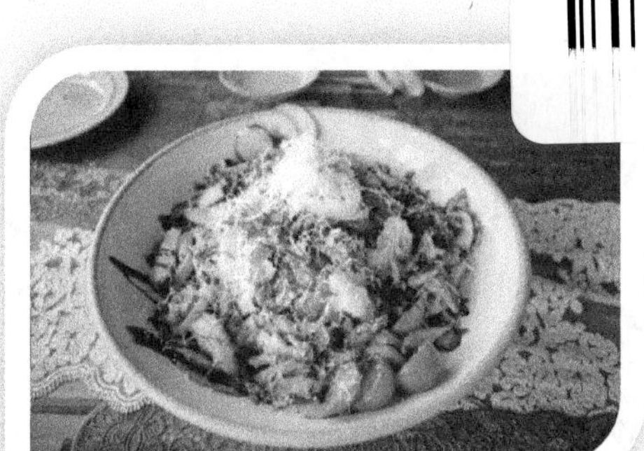

Anti- Inflammatory recipe guide for Hypertension free lifestyle

DR.CATHERINE THOMAS

Text Copyright© 2024 by Dr. Catherine Thomas

All rights reserved worldwide No part of this publication may be republished in any form or by any means, including photocopying, scanning or otherwise without prior written permission to the copyright holder.

This book contains nonfictional content. The views expressed are those of the author and do not necessarily represent those of the publisher. In addition, the publisher declaims any responsibility for them.

TABLE OF CONTENT

INTRODUCTION

Welcome to the **"THE ULTIMATE DASH Diet Cookbook for Seniors"**! I am Dr. Catherine Thomas, a nutritionist with years of experience dedicated to helping individuals achieve optimal health through mindful eating. Over the years, I have seen firsthand the transformative power of a balanced diet, particularly for seniors who face unique health challenges as they age.

The DASH (Dietary Approaches to Stop Hypertension) diet is a well-researched eating plan designed to combat high blood pressure and promote heart health. It emphasizes the consumption of fruits, vegetables, whole grains, lean proteins, and low-fat dairy while limiting salt, red meat, and added sugars. This diet not only helps manage hypertension but also supports overall well-being, making it an excellent choice for seniors.

A Path to Better Health

As we age, our bodies undergo various changes that can impact our health. Many seniors are at a higher risk of developing chronic conditions such as hypertension, heart disease, diabetes, and inflammation-related disorders. The DASH diet is specifically designed to address these issues by providing a nutrient-dense, anti-inflammatory approach to eating.

Hypertension and Heart Health: Hypertension, or high blood pressure, is a common issue among seniors and a major risk factor for heart disease and stroke. The DASH diet has been shown to significantly reduce blood pressure levels, thanks to its focus on potassium-rich foods like fruits and vegetables, which help counteract the effects of sodium.

Diabetes Management: For seniors with diabetes or at risk of developing it, the DASH diet offers a balanced way to manage blood sugar levels. Its emphasis on whole grains, lean proteins, and healthy fats helps maintain steady glucose levels and reduces the risk of insulin resistance.

Inflammation and Chronic Disease: Chronic inflammation is at the root of many age-related diseases, including arthritis, Alzheimer's, and certain cancers. The anti-inflammatory properties of the DASH diet, derived from its rich array of antioxidants and phytochemicals found in plant-based foods, help combat inflammation and promote long-term health.

A Personal Note

Throughout my career, I have been inspired by the stories of countless seniors who have turned their health around by adopting the DASH diet. One such story is of my dear friend, Margaret. At 72, Margaret was struggling with high blood pressure and arthritis. After transitioning to the DASH diet, she not only saw her blood pressure drop but also experienced reduced joint pain and increased energy levels. Her journey reaffirmed my belief in the power of nutrition to heal and rejuvenate.

In this cookbook, you will find a collection of nutritious and flavorful anti-inflammatory recipes designed to help you embrace the DASH diet and enhance your health. Each recipe is crafted to provide maximum nutritional benefit while delighting your taste buds. I invite you to embark on this journey to better health with me, one delicious meal at a time

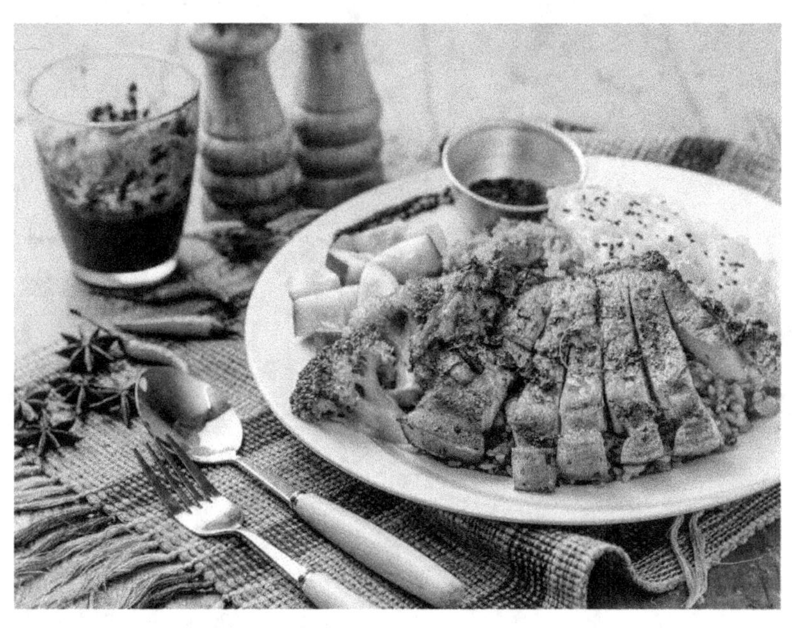

Part 1:

Understanding the DASH Diet

The Dietary Approaches to Stop Hypertension (DASH) diet is a well-established and research-backed eating plan designed to combat high blood pressure (hypertension) and promote overall heart health. Developed in the 1990s with support from the National Institutes of Health (NIH), the DASH diet emphasizes nutrient-dense foods that are naturally low in sodium and high in potassium, magnesium, and calcium—key minerals that help regulate blood pressure.

Types of the DASH Diet

The DASH diet comes in two primary variations: the Standard DASH Diet and the Lower Sodium DASH Diet.

1. **Standard DASH Diet:** This version allows up to 2,300 milligrams (mg) of sodium per day, aligning with the dietary guidelines for reducing the risk of hypertension and maintaining heart health.

2. **Lower Sodium DASH Diet:** For individuals needing a more stringent reduction in sodium intake, this version caps sodium consumption at 1,500 mg per day. This approach is particularly beneficial for those with higher blood pressure or salt sensitivity.

Causes of Hypertension Addressed by the DASH Diet

Hypertension can develop due to a combination of factors, many of which are addressed by the DASH diet:

Dietary Factors: High sodium intake is a well-known contributor to hypertension. The DASH diet mitigates this risk by encouraging foods rich in potassium, magnesium, and calcium, which help balance blood pressure.

Obesity and Overweight: Excess body weight strains the heart and blood vessels, leading to hypertension. The DASH diet promotes weight loss and maintenance through balanced, low-calorie, nutrient-dense meals.

Lack of Physical Activity: Sedentary lifestyles increase the risk of hypertension. Although primarily a dietary plan, the DASH diet works best when combined with regular physical activity.

Excessive Alcohol Consumption: Alcohol can raise blood pressure and contribute to weight gain. The DASH diet advises moderation in alcohol intake.

Hypertension is often called the "silent killer" because it typically has no noticeable symptoms until significant damage has occurred. However, in some cases, individuals may experience:

Headaches: Severe headaches can be a sign of very high blood pressure.

Shortness of Breath: Difficulty breathing may occur due to the strain on the heart.

Nosebleeds: Frequent nosebleeds can be associated with high blood pressure.

Chest Pain: Chest discomfort or pain might indicate heart-related complications from hypertension.

Vision Problems: Blurred vision or vision loss can occur if high blood pressure damages the blood vessels in the eyes.

Preventive Measures and the Role of the DASH Diet

The DASH diet is not only a treatment but also a preventive measure against hypertension and related health issues. Here are key preventive strategies:

1. **Adopt the DASH Diet Early**: Starting the DASH diet early, even before the onset of hypertension, can help prevent the condition. The diet's emphasis on fruits, vegetables, whole grains, lean proteins, and low-fat dairy provides essential nutrients that support cardiovascular health.

2. **Maintain a Healthy Weight**: The DASH diet's balanced approach aids in weight management, which is crucial for preventing hypertension. Reducing excess weight alleviates pressure on the cardiovascular system.

3. **Reduce Sodium Intake**: Limiting sodium is a cornerstone of the DASH diet. Using herbs and spices instead of salt to flavor foods can help lower blood pressure.

4. **Increase Physical Activity**: Regular exercise complements the DASH diet. Aim for at least 150 minutes of moderate aerobic activity or 75 minutes of vigorous activity each week.

5. **Limit Alcohol and Avoid Tobacco**: Moderation in alcohol consumption and avoiding tobacco products are essential for maintaining healthy blood pressure levels.

6. **Monitor Blood Pressure**: Regular monitoring of blood pressure can help detect hypertension early and manage it effectively with dietary and lifestyle changes.

The DASH diet is a powerful tool for preventing and managing hypertension, offering a comprehensive approach to nutrition that supports heart health and overall well-being. By adopting this diet, along with other healthy lifestyle practices, seniors can significantly reduce their risk of hypertension and enjoy a higher quality of life.

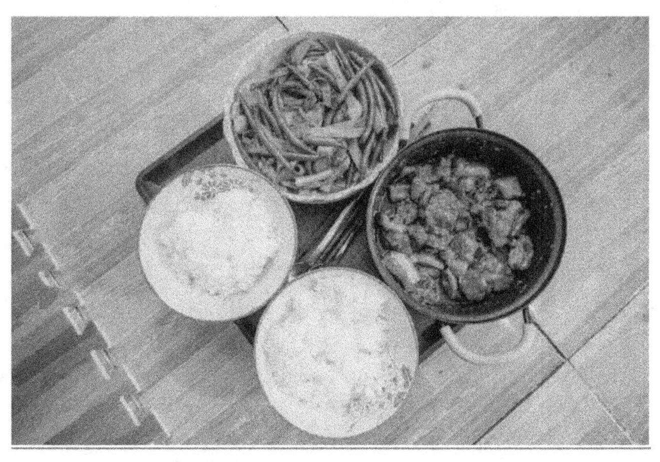

Part 2:

Foods to Eat and Avoid on the DASH Diet for Optimum Health

The DASH (Dietary Approaches to Stop Hypertension) diet is designed to promote heart health and reduce high blood pressure through a balanced and nutritious eating plan. To achieve optimal health on the DASH diet, it's essential to focus on specific foods to include and avoid. Here's a detailed guide on what to eat and what to avoid.

Foods to Eat

1. **Fruits and Vegetables:**

   Fruits: Aim for 4-5 servings of fruits per day. Fresh, frozen, or canned fruits without added sugar are excellent choices. Berries, apples, oranges, bananas, and pears are rich in vitamins, minerals, and fiber.

   Vegetables: Aim for 4-5 servings of vegetables per day. Leafy greens, tomatoes, carrots, and broccoli are nutrient-dense and provide essential vitamins, minerals, and fiber.

2. **Whole Grains**:

Include 6-8 servings of whole grains daily. Whole grains such as brown rice, quinoa, whole wheat bread, and oatmeal are rich in fiber, which helps maintain a healthy digestive system and regulate blood sugar levels.

3. **Lean Proteins**:

Aim for 2 or fewer servings of lean meat, poultry, or fish per day. Choose lean cuts of meat, skinless poultry, and fish like salmon, tuna, and mackerel, which are high in omega-3 fatty acids.

Plant-Based Proteins: Incorporate beans, lentils, tofu, and nuts for a protein boost. These are excellent alternatives to meat and provide additional fiber and nutrients.

4. **Low-Fat Dairy**:

Consume 2-3 servings of low-fat or fat-free dairy products daily. Options include milk, yogurt, and cheese. These provide calcium, vitamin D, and protein without the added saturated fat.

5. **Nuts, Seeds, and Legumes:**

Include 4-5 servings of nuts, seeds, and legumes per week. Almonds, walnuts, sunflower seeds, and legumes like lentils and chickpeas offer healthy fats, protein, and fiber.

6. **Healthy Fats:**

Use healthy fats in moderation. Opt for olive oil, avocado, and fatty fish. These fats are beneficial for heart health and help reduce inflammation.

7. **Herbs and Spices:**

Use herbs and spices to flavor foods instead of salt. Basil, oregano, rosemary, garlic, and turmeric add flavor and additional health benefits.

Foods to Avoid

1. **High-Sodium Foods:**

Limit sodium intake to less than 2,300 milligrams per day, or 1,500 milligrams for those with hypertension. Avoid processed foods, canned soups, salty snacks, and restaurant meals, which are typically high in sodium.

2. **Sugary Foods and Beverages:**

Avoid foods and drinks with added sugars, such as soda, candy, pastries, and desserts. These contribute to weight gain and increase the risk of heart disease and diabetes.

3. **Red and Processed Meats:**

Limit consumption of red meat and avoid processed meats like bacon, sausage, and deli meats. These are high in saturated fats and sodium, which can raise blood pressure and cholesterol levels.

4. **Full-Fat Dairy:**

Avoid full-fat dairy products, such as whole milk, full-fat cheese, and butter. These are high in saturated fats, which can increase cholesterol levels and heart disease risk.

5. **Refined Grains:**

Limit refined grains, such as white bread, white rice, and pastries. These have been stripped of essential nutrients and fiber, leading to spikes in blood sugar levels.

6. **Fried Foods**:

> Avoid fried foods, which are high in unhealthy fats and calories. Instead, opt for baked, grilled, or steamed options.

7. **Alcohol**:

> Limit alcohol consumption to no more than one drink per day for women and two drinks per day for men. Excessive alcohol intake can raise blood pressure and contribute to other health issues.

Following the DASH diet involves making conscious food choices to include nutrient-rich foods while avoiding those that can harm your health. By focusing on fruits, vegetables, whole grains, lean proteins, low-fat dairy, nuts, seeds, and healthy fats, and by minimizing high-sodium, sugary, and fatty foods, you can achieve optimal health and effectively manage blood pressure. This balanced approach to eating not only supports cardiovascular health but also enhances overall well-being.

Here's a 7 day sample DASH diet meal plan designed to provide balanced, nutritious, and flavorful meals while helping to manage blood pressure and promote overall health. Each day includes breakfast, lunch, dinner, and snacks.

Day 1

Breakfast:

Oatmeal with fresh berries and a sprinkle of chia seeds

Low-fat milk

Lunch:

Quinoa salad with mixed vegetables, chickpeas, and a lemon-tahini dressing

An apple

Dinner:

Grilled salmon

Steamed broccoli

Brown rice

Snacks:

Carrot sticks with hummus

A handful of almonds

Day 2

Breakfast:

Greek yogurt with honey and sliced almonds

A banana

Lunch:

Whole wheat wrap with turkey, lettuce, tomato, and avocado

A side of mixed greens with balsamic vinaigrette

Dinner:

Stir-fried tofu with mixed vegetables

Quinoa

Snacks:

A pear

Low-fat string cheese

Day 3

Breakfast:

Whole grain toast with avocado and a poached egg

A grapefruit

Lunch:

Lentil soup

Whole grain roll

Dinner:

Baked chicken breast

Roasted sweet potatoes

Green beans

Snacks:

Sliced cucumber with tzatziki

A handful of walnuts

Breakfast:

Smoothie with spinach, banana, berries, and almond milk

Lunch:

Tuna salad with mixed greens, cherry tomatoes, and olive oil dressing

Whole grain crackers

Dinner:

Spaghetti with whole wheat pasta, marinara sauce, and turkey meatballs

Steamed zucchini

Snacks:

An orange

Low-fat cottage cheese

Day 5

Breakfast:

Whole grain cereal with low-fat milk and sliced strawberries

Lunch:

Black bean and corn salad with lime dressing

Whole grain tortilla chips

Dinner:

Baked cod

Quinoa pilaf

Steamed asparagus

Snacks:

A handful of baby carrots

An apple with peanut butter

Day 6

Breakfast:

Scrambled eggs with spinach and tomatoes

Whole grain toast

Lunch:

Grilled chicken salad with mixed greens, cucumber, and a light vinaigrette

A small piece of whole grain bread

Dinner:

Vegetable stir-fry with tofu

Brown rice

Snacks:

A peach

A handful of almonds

Day 7

Breakfast:

Greek yogurt with granola and fresh fruit

Lunch:

Whole wheat pita with hummus, cucumber, and bell peppers

A side salad

Dinner:

Baked salmon

Steamed broccoli

Couscous

Snacks:

Sliced bell peppers with guacamole

A handful of mixed nuts

Part 3:

Breakfast:

1. Berry Oatmeal

Ingredients:

1 cup rolled oats

2 cups low-fat milk or water

1/2 cup fresh blueberries

1/2 cup fresh strawberries, sliced

1 tablespoon chia seeds

1 teaspoon honey (optional)

Preparation:

1. In a pot, bring the milk or water to a boil.

2. Add oats and reduce heat to a simmer, cooking for 5-7 minutes.

3. Stir in the berries and chia seeds.

4. Drizzle with honey if desired.

Nutritional Value:

Calories: 300

Protein: 10g

Carbohydrates: 55g

Fat: 5g

Fiber: 10g

Cooking Time: 10 minutes

2. Avocado Toast with Egg

Ingredients:

1 slice whole grain bread

1/2 avocado, mashed

1 large egg

Salt and pepper to taste

1 teaspoon olive oil

Preparation:

1. Toast the bread.

2. Spread mashed avocado on the toast.

3. Heat olive oil in a pan over medium heat and cook the egg sunny-side up.

4. Place the egg on top of the avocado toast and season with salt and pepper.

Nutritional Value:

Calories: 280

Protein: 10g

Carbohydrates: 22g

Fat: 18g

Fiber: 7g

Cooking Time: 10 minutes

3. Greek Yogurt Parfait

Ingredients:

1 cup Greek yogurt

1/2 cup granola (low sugar)

1/2 cup mixed berries (blueberries, raspberries, strawberries)

1 tablespoon honey

Preparation:

1. Layer Greek yogurt, granola, and mixed berries in a bowl or glass.

2. Drizzle with honey.

Nutritional Value:

Calories: 350

Protein: 20g

Carbohydrates: 55g

Fat: 7g

Fiber: 5g

Cooking Time: 5 minutes

4. Spinach and Feta Omelette

Ingredients:

2 large eggs

1/2 cup fresh spinach, chopped

1/4 cup feta cheese, crumbled

1 teaspoon olive oil

Salt and pepper to taste

Preparation:

1. Whisk the eggs in a bowl and season with salt and pepper.

2. Heat olive oil in a non-stick pan over medium heat.

3. Add spinach and sauté until wilted.

4. Pour eggs into the pan and cook until they start to set.

5. Sprinkle feta cheese on one half of the omelette.

6. Fold the omelette and cook for another 1-2 minutes.

Nutritional Value:

Calories: 250

Protein: 18g

Carbohydrates: 4g

Fat: 18g

Fiber: 1g

Cooking Time: 10 minutes

5. Banana Almond Smoothie

Ingredients:

1 banana

1 cup almond milk (unsweetened)

1 tablespoon almond butter

1 teaspoon honey

1/2 teaspoon cinnamon

Preparation:

1. Combine all ingredients in a blender.

2. Blend until smooth.

Nutritional Value:

Calories: 250

Protein: 4g

Carbohydrates: 38g

Fat: 10g

Fiber: 4g

Cooking Time: 5 minutes

6. Whole Grain Pancakes

Ingredients:

1 cup whole wheat flour

1 tablespoon baking powder

1 cup low-fat milk

1 large egg

1 tablespoon olive oil

1 tablespoon honey

Preparation:

1. In a bowl, mix flour and baking powder.

2. In another bowl, whisk together milk, egg, olive oil, and honey.

3. Combine wet and dry ingredients and stir until smooth.

4. Heat a non-stick pan over medium heat and pour 1/4 cup batter for each pancake.

5. Cook until bubbles form, then flip and cook another 1-2 minutes.

Nutritional Value:

Calories: 300 (per serving)

Protein: 10g

Carbohydrates: 50g

Fat: 8g

Fiber: 5g   **Cooking Time: 15 minutes**

7. Chia Seed Pudding

Ingredients:

1/4 cup chia seeds

1 cup almond milk

1 tablespoon honey

1/2 teaspoon vanilla extract

Fresh fruit for topping

Preparation:

1. Mix chia seeds, almond milk, honey, and vanilla extract in a bowl.

2. Refrigerate for at least 4 hours or overnight.

3. Top with fresh fruit before serving.

Nutritional Value:

Calories: 250

Protein: 5g

Carbohydrates: 30g

Fat: 12g

Fiber: 10g

Cooking Time: 5 minutes (plus chilling time)

8. Peanut Butter Banana Toast

Ingredients:

1 slice whole grain bread

1 tablespoon peanut butter

1/2 banana, sliced

1 teaspoon chia seeds

Preparation:

1. Toast the bread.

2. Spread peanut butter on the toast.

3. Arrange banana slices on top and sprinkle with chia seeds.

Nutritional Value:

Calories: 280

Protein: 8g

Carbohydrates: 30g

Fat: 14g

Fiber: 6g

Cooking Time: 5 minutes

9. Veggie Breakfast Burrito

Ingredients:

1 whole wheat tortilla

2 large eggs

1/4 cup black beans

1/4 cup diced tomatoes

1/4 cup diced bell peppers

1/4 cup shredded low-fat cheese

1 teaspoon olive oil

Salt and pepper to taste

Preparation:

1. Whisk the eggs in a bowl and season with salt and pepper.

2. Heat olive oil in a non-stick pan over medium heat.

3. Sauté the bell peppers and tomatoes until soft.

4. Add eggs and black beans, and scramble until cooked.

5. Place the mixture on the tortilla, sprinkle with cheese, and roll up.

Nutritional Value:

Calories: 350

Protein: 20g

Carbohydrates: 35g

Fat: 15g

Fiber: 8g

Cooking Time: 10 minutes

10. Apple Cinnamon Quinoa
Ingredients:

1/2 cup quinoa

1 cup water

1/2 apple, diced

1/4 teaspoon cinnamon

1 tablespoon chopped walnuts

1 teaspoon honey

Preparation:

1. Rinse quinoa under cold water.

2. In a pot, combine quinoa and water, bring to a boil.

3. Reduce heat and simmer for 15 minutes, until water is absorbed.

4. Stir in diced apple, cinnamon, walnuts, and honey.

Nutritional Value:

Calories: 300

Protein: 8g

Carbohydrates: 55g

Fat: 8g

Fiber: 6g

Cooking Time: 20 minutes

1. Quinoa and Black Bean Salad

Ingredients:

1 cup quinoa, cooked

1 can (15 oz) black beans, rinsed and drained

1 cup cherry tomatoes, halved

1 avocado, diced

1/4 cup red onion, finely chopped

1/4 cup cilantro, chopped

2 tablespoons olive oil

1 tablespoon lime juice

Salt and pepper to taste

Preparation:

1. Combine quinoa, black beans, cherry tomatoes, avocado, red onion, and cilantro in a large bowl.

2. In a small bowl, whisk together olive oil, lime juice, salt, and pepper.

3. Pour dressing over the salad and toss to combine.

Nutritional Value:

Calories: 350

Protein: 12g

Carbohydrates: 45g

Fat: 15g

Fiber: 12g

Cooking Time: 20 minutes

2. Grilled Chicken and Veggie Wrap

Ingredients:

1 whole wheat tortilla

1 grilled chicken breast, sliced

1/2 cup mixed greens

1/4 cup shredded carrots

1/4 cup sliced bell peppers

2 tablespoons hummus

Salt and pepper to taste

Preparation:

1. Spread hummus on the whole wheat tortilla.

2. Layer grilled chicken, mixed greens, carrots, and bell peppers.

3. Season with salt and pepper.

4. Roll up the tortilla and slice in half.

Nutritional Value:

Calories: 300

Protein: 25g

Carbohydrates: 35g

Fat: 8g

Fiber: 8g

Cooking Time: 15 minutes

3. Lentil Soup

Ingredients:

1 cup lentils, rinsed

1 carrot, diced

1 celery stalk, diced

1 small onion, diced

2 cloves garlic, minced

1 can (15 oz) diced tomatoes

4 cups low-sodium vegetable broth

1 teaspoon cumin

1 teaspoon paprika

2 tablespoons olive oil

Salt and pepper to taste

Preparation:

1. Heat olive oil in a large pot over medium heat.

2. Add carrot, celery, and onion, and sauté until softened, about 5 minutes.

3. Add garlic, cumin, and paprika, and cook for another minute.

4. Stir in lentils, diced tomatoes, and vegetable broth.

5. Bring to a boil, then reduce heat and simmer for 25-30 minutes, until lentils are tender.

6. Season with salt and pepper.

Nutritional Value:

Calories: 250

Protein: 15g

Carbohydrates: 40g

Fat: 6g

Fiber: 15g

Cooking Time: 35 minutes

4. Spinach and Feta Stuffed Peppers

Ingredients:

2 bell peppers, halved and seeds removed

1 cup cooked quinoa

1 cup fresh spinach, chopped

1/4 cup feta cheese, crumbled

1/4 cup diced tomatoes

1 tablespoon olive oil

Salt and pepper to taste

Preparation:

1. Preheat oven to 375°F (190°C).

2. In a bowl, mix cooked quinoa, spinach, feta cheese, diced tomatoes, olive oil, salt, and pepper.

3. Stuff the bell pepper halves with the quinoa mixture.

4. Place stuffed peppers in a baking dish and bake for 25-30 minutes, until peppers are tender.

Nutritional Value:

Calories: 250

Protein: 8g

Carbohydrates: 35g

Fat: 10g

Fiber: 8g   **Cooking Time: 30 minutes**

5. Turkey and Avocado Salad

Ingredients:

2 cups mixed greens

4 oz cooked turkey breast, sliced

1/2 avocado, diced

1/2 cup cherry tomatoes, halved

1/4 cup cucumber, sliced

1 tablespoon olive oil

1 tablespoon balsamic vinegar

Salt and pepper to taste

Preparation:

1. In a large bowl, combine mixed greens, turkey, avocado, cherry tomatoes, and cucumber.

2. In a small bowl, whisk together olive oil, balsamic vinegar, salt, and pepper.

3. Pour dressing over the salad and toss to combine.

Nutritional Value:

Calories: 300

Protein: 25g

Carbohydrates: 15g

Fat: 18g

Fiber: 6g

Cooking Time: 10 minutes

6. Chickpea and Veggie Stir-Fry

Ingredients:

1 can (15 oz) chickpeas, rinsed and drained

1 cup broccoli florets

1 red bell pepper, sliced

1 carrot, sliced

2 tablespoons soy sauce (low sodium)

1 tablespoon olive oil

1 teaspoon ginger, minced

2 cloves garlic, minced

1 cup cooked brown rice

Preparation:

1. Heat olive oil in a pan over medium heat.

2. Add garlic and ginger, and sauté for 1 minute.

3. Add broccoli, bell pepper, and carrot, and cook for 5-7 minutes until tender.

4. Stir in chickpeas and soy sauce, and cook for another 3-4 minutes.

5. Serve over cooked brown rice.

Nutritional Value:

Calories: 350

Protein: 12g

Carbohydrates: 55g

Fat: 10g

Fiber: 10g

Cooking Time: 20 minutes

7. Tuna and White Bean Salad

Ingredients:

1 can (5 oz) tuna in water, drained

1 can (15 oz) white beans, rinsed and drained

1/4 cup red onion, finely chopped

1/4 cup celery, diced

2 tablespoons olive oil

1 tablespoon lemon juice

1 teaspoon Dijon mustard

Salt and pepper to taste

Preparation:

1. In a large bowl, combine tuna, white beans, red onion, and celery.

2. In a small bowl, whisk together olive oil, lemon juice, Dijon mustard, salt, and pepper.

3. Pour dressing over the salad and toss to combine.

Nutritional Value:

Calories: 300

Protein: 25g

Carbohydrates: 25g

Fat: 12g

Fiber: 8g

Cooking Time: 10 minutes

8. Mediterranean Chickpea Salad

Ingredients:

1 can (15 oz) chickpeas, rinsed and drained

1/2 cup cherry tomatoes, halved

1/2 cup cucumber, diced

1/4 cup red onion, finely chopped

1/4 cup Kalamata olives, sliced

2 tablespoons feta cheese, crumbled

2 tablespoons olive oil

1 tablespoon red wine vinegar

1 teaspoon oregano

Salt and pepper to taste

Preparation:

1. In a large bowl, combine chickpeas, cherry tomatoes, cucumber, red onion, and olives.

2. In a small bowl, whisk together olive oil, red wine vinegar, oregano, salt, and pepper.

3. Pour dressing over the salad and toss to combine.

4. Sprinkle feta cheese on top.

Nutritional Value:

Calories: 300

Protein: 10g

Carbohydrates: 30g

Fat: 15g

Fiber: 8g

Cooking Time: 10 minutes

9. Vegetable and Hummus Sandwich

Ingredients:

2 slices whole grain bread

2 tablespoons hummus

1/2 cup spinach leaves

1/4 cup cucumber slices

1/4 cup shredded carrots

1/4 cup bell pepper slices

Preparation:

1. Spread hummus on both slices of whole grain bread.

2. Layer spinach, cucumber, shredded carrots, and bell pepper on one slice of bread.

3. Top with the other slice of bread and slice in half.

Nutritional Value:

Calories: 250

Protein: 8g

Carbohydrates: 40g

Fat: 8g

Fiber: 8g

Cooking Time: 5 minutes

10. Shrimp and Avocado Salad

Ingredients:

2 cups mixed greens

1/2 cup cooked shrimp

1/2 avocado, diced

1/4 cup cherry tomatoes, halved

1/4 cup cucumber, sliced

2 tablespoons olive oil

1 tablespoon lemon juice

Salt and pepper to taste

Preparation:

1. In a large bowl, combine mixed greens, shrimp, avocado, cherry tomatoes, and cucumber.

2. In a small bowl, whisk together olive oil, lemon juice, salt, and pepper.

3. Pour dressing over the salad and toss to combine.

Nutritional Value:

Calories: 300

Protein: 15g

Carbohydrates: 15g

Fat: 20g

Fiber: 6g

Cooking Time: 10 minutes

Dinner:

1. Baked Salmon with Asparagus

Ingredients:

4 salmon fillets (6 oz each)

1 bunch asparagus, trimmed

2 tablespoons olive oil

1 lemon, sliced

2 cloves garlic, minced

Salt and pepper to taste

Preparation:

1. Preheat oven to 400°F (200°C).

2. Place salmon fillets and asparagus on a baking sheet.

3. Drizzle with olive oil and sprinkle with garlic, salt, and pepper.

4. Arrange lemon slices on top of salmon.

5. Bake for 15-20 minutes, until salmon is cooked through.

Nutritional Value:

Calories: 400

Protein: 35g

Carbohydrates: 10g

Fat: 25g

Fiber: 4g   **Cooking Time: 25 minutes**

2. Quinoa-Stuffed Bell Peppers

Ingredients:

4 bell peppers, halved and seeds removed

1 cup cooked quinoa

1 cup black beans, rinsed and drained

1 cup corn kernels

1 cup diced tomatoes

1/4 cup chopped cilantro

1 teaspoon cumin

1 teaspoon paprika

Salt and pepper to taste

Preparation:

1. Preheat oven to 375°F (190°C).

2. In a bowl, combine cooked quinoa, black beans, corn, tomatoes, cilantro, cumin, paprika, salt, and pepper.

3. Stuff bell pepper halves with quinoa mixture.

4. Place stuffed peppers in a baking dish and bake for 25-30 minutes.

Nutritional Value:

Calories: 300

Protein: 12g

Carbohydrates: 50g

Fat: 5g

Fiber: 12g

Cooking Time: 35 minutes

3. Lemon Herb Chicken

Ingredients:

4 boneless, skinless chicken breasts (6 oz each)

2 tablespoons olive oil

2 tablespoons lemon juice

1 tablespoon chopped fresh rosemary

1 tablespoon chopped fresh thyme

2 cloves garlic, minced

Salt and pepper to taste

Preparation:

1. In a bowl, mix olive oil, lemon juice, rosemary, thyme, garlic, salt, and pepper.

2. Add chicken breasts and marinate for at least 30 minutes.

3. Preheat grill or grill pan to medium-high heat.

4. Grill chicken for 6-7 minutes on each side, until fully cooked.

Nutritional Value:

Calories: 300

Protein: 35g

Carbohydrates: 2g

Fat: 16g

Fiber: 0g

Cooking Time: 20 minutes (plus marinating time)

4. Veggie Stir-Fry with Tofu

Ingredients:

1 block (14 oz) firm tofu, drained and cubed

1 cup broccoli florets

1 red bell pepper, sliced

1 carrot, julienned

2 tablespoons soy sauce (low sodium)

1 tablespoon olive oil

2 cloves garlic, minced

1 teaspoon ginger, minced

1 cup cooked brown rice

Preparation:

1. Heat olive oil in a pan over medium heat.

2. Add garlic and ginger, and sauté for 1 minute.

3. Add tofu and cook until golden brown, about 5-7 minutes.

4. Add broccoli, bell pepper, and carrot, and cook for another 5-7 minutes.

5. Stir in soy sauce and cook for another 2 minutes.

6. Serve over cooked brown rice.

Nutritional Value:

Calories: 350

Protein: 18g

Carbohydrates: 45g

Fat: 12g

Fiber: 8g

Cooking Time: 20 minutes

5. Spaghetti Squash Primavera

Ingredients:

1 spaghetti squash

1 cup cherry tomatoes, halved

1 zucchini, sliced

1 yellow squash, sliced

1/4 cup grated Parmesan cheese

2 tablespoons olive oil

2 cloves garlic, minced

Salt and pepper to taste

Preparation:

1. Preheat oven to 375°F (190°C).

2. Cut spaghetti squash in half, remove seeds, and place cut-side down on a baking sheet.

3. Bake for 40-45 minutes, until tender.

4. Use a fork to scrape out spaghetti squash strands.

5. In a large pan, heat olive oil over medium heat.

6. Add garlic and sauté for 1 minute.

7. Add cherry tomatoes, zucchini, and yellow squash, and cook for 5-7 minutes.

8. Stir in spaghetti squash strands and Parmesan cheese.

9. Season with salt and pepper.

Nutritional Value:

Calories: 250

Protein: 8g

Carbohydrates: 30g

Fat: 12g

Fiber: 6g

Cooking Time: 50 minutes

6. Baked Cod with Tomatoes and Olives

Ingredients:

4 cod fillets (6 oz each)

1 cup cherry tomatoes, halved

1/4 cup Kalamata olives, sliced

2 tablespoons olive oil

2 cloves garlic, minced

1 tablespoon lemon juice

Salt and pepper to taste

Preparation:

1. Preheat oven to 375°F (190°C).

2. Place cod fillets in a baking dish.

3. In a bowl, mix cherry tomatoes, olives, olive oil, garlic, lemon juice, salt, and pepper.

4. Spoon tomato mixture over cod fillets.

5. Bake for 20-25 minutes, until fish is cooked through.

Nutritional Value:

Calories: 300

Protein: 35g

Carbohydrates: 10g

Fat: 12g

Fiber: 3g   **Cooking Time: 30 minutes**

7. Turkey and Sweet Potato Skillet

Ingredients:

1 lb ground turkey

2 sweet potatoes, diced

1 red bell pepper, diced

1 green bell pepper, diced

1 onion, diced

2 tablespoons olive oil

2 cloves garlic, minced

1 teaspoon paprika

Salt and pepper to taste

Preparation:

1. Heat olive oil in a large skillet over medium heat.

2. Add onion and garlic, and sauté for 3-4 minutes.

3. Add ground turkey and cook until browned, about 5-7 minutes.

4. Add sweet potatoes, bell peppers, paprika, salt, and pepper.

5. Cover and cook for 10-15 minutes, until sweet potatoes are tender.

Nutritional Value:

Calories: 350

Protein: 25g

Carbohydrates: 35g

Fat: 12g

Fiber: 6g

Cooking Time: 25 minutes

8. Chickpea and Spinach Curry

Ingredients:

1 can (15 oz) chickpeas, rinsed and drained

1 can (14 oz) diced tomatoes

4 cups fresh spinach

1 onion, diced

2 cloves garlic, minced

1 tablespoon olive oil

1 tablespoon curry powder

1 teaspoon cumin

1 cup cooked brown rice

Preparation:

1. Heat olive oil in a large pan over medium heat.

2. Add onion and garlic, and sauté for 3-4 minutes.

3. Stir in curry powder and cumin, and cook for another minute.

4. Add chickpeas and diced tomatoes, and simmer for 10 minutes.

5. Stir in spinach and cook until wilted.

6. Serve over cooked brown rice.

Nutritional Value:

Calories: 300

Protein: 12g

Carbohydrates: 50g

Fat: 8g

Fiber: 10g

Cooking Time: 20 minutes

9. Grilled Vegetable Kebabs

Ingredients:

1 zucchini, sliced

1 yellow squash, sliced

1 red bell pepper, cut into chunks

1 green bell pepper, cut into chunks

1 red onion, cut into chunks

2 tablespoons olive oil

1 tablespoon balsamic vinegar

Salt and pepper to taste

Wooden skewers, soaked in water

Preparation:

1. Preheat grill to medium-high heat.

2. Thread vegetables onto skewers.

3. In a small bowl, mix olive oil, balsamic vinegar, salt, and pepper.

4. Brush vegetable skewers with the oil mixture.

5. Grill for 10-15 minutes, turning occasionally, until vegetables are tender and slightly charred.

Nutritional Value:

Calories: 150

Protein: 4g

Carbohydrates: 20g

Fat: 8g

Fiber: 6g   **Cooking Time: 20 minutes**

10. Chicken and Vegetable Stir-Fry

Ingredients:

1 lb chicken breast, sliced

1 cup broccoli florets

1 red bell pepper, sliced

1 carrot, julienned

2 tablespoons soy sauce (low sodium)

2 tablespoons olive oil

2 cloves garlic, minced

1 teaspoon ginger, minced

1 cup cooked brown rice

Preparation:

1. Heat olive oil in a large pan over medium heat.

2. Add garlic and ginger, and sauté for 1 minute.

3. Add chicken and cook until browned, about 5-7 minutes.

4. Add broccoli, bell pepper, and carrot, and cook for another 5-7 minutes.

5. Stir in soy sauce and cook for another 2 minutes.

6. Serve over cooked brown rice.

Nutritional Value:

Calories: 350

Protein: 30g

Carbohydrates: 40g

Fat: 10g

Fiber: 6g

Cooking Time: 20 minutes

Snacks:

1. Apple Slices with Almond Butter

Ingredients:

1 apple, sliced

2 tablespoons almond butter

Preparation:

1. Core and slice the apple.

2. Serve apple slices with almond butter for dipping.

Nutritional Value:

Calories: 200

Protein: 4g

Carbohydrates: 28g

Fat: 9g

Fiber: 6g

Cooking Time: 5 minutes

2. Greek Yogurt with Berries

Ingredients:

1 cup plain Greek yogurt

1/2 cup mixed berries (strawberries, blueberries, raspberries)

1 tablespoon honey

Preparation:

1. Place Greek yogurt in a bowl.

2. Top with mixed berries and drizzle with honey.

Nutritional Value:

Calories: 180

Protein: 14g

Carbohydrates: 22g

Fat: 4g

Fiber: 3g

Cooking Time: 5 minutes

3. Veggie Sticks with Hummus

Ingredients:

1 cup carrot sticks

1 cup cucumber sticks

1 cup celery sticks

1/4 cup hummus

Preparation:

1. Arrange carrot, cucumber, and celery sticks on a plate.

2. Serve with hummus for dipping.

Nutritional Value:

Calories: 150

Protein: 4g

Carbohydrates: 18g

Fat: 8g

Fiber: 6g

Cooking Time: 5 minutes

4. Cottage Cheese with Pineapple

Ingredients:

1 cup low-fat cottage cheese

1/2 cup pineapple chunks (fresh or canned in juice)

Preparation:

1. Place cottage cheese in a bowl.

2. Top with pineapple chunks.

Nutritional Value:

Calories: 180

Protein: 14g

Carbohydrates: 20g

Fat: 4g

Fiber: 2g

Cooking Time: 5 minutes

5. Roasted Chickpeas

Ingredients:

1 can (15 oz) chickpeas, rinsed and drained

1 tablespoon olive oil

1 teaspoon paprika

1/2 teaspoon garlic powder

Salt to taste

Preparation:

1. Preheat oven to 400°F (200°C).

2. Pat chickpeas dry with a paper towel.

3. Toss chickpeas with olive oil, paprika, garlic powder, and salt.

4. Spread chickpeas on a baking sheet and bake for 20-25 minutes, until crispy.

Nutritional Value:

Calories: 180

Protein: 6g

Carbohydrates: 24g

Fat: 7g

Fiber: 6g

Cooking Time: 30 minutes

6. Almonds and Dark Chocolate

Ingredients:

1/4 cup raw almonds

1 oz dark chocolate (70% cocoa or higher)

Preparation:

1. Portion out almonds and dark chocolate.

Nutritional Value:

Calories: 220

Protein: 5g

Carbohydrates: 18g

Fat: 15g

Fiber: 5g

Cooking Time: 2 minutes

7. Avocado Toast

Ingredients:

1 slice whole grain bread

1/2 avocado, mashed

Salt and pepper to taste

Red pepper flakes (optional)

Preparation:

1. Toast the whole grain bread.

2. Spread mashed avocado on toast.

3. Season with salt, pepper, and red pepper flakes if desired.

Nutritional Value:

Calories: 200

Protein: 4g

Carbohydrates: 24g

Fat: 12g

Fiber: 8g

Cooking Time: 5 minutes

8. Banana and Peanut Butter

Ingredients:

1 banana

1 tablespoon peanut butter

Preparation:

1. Peel the banana and cut it into slices.

2. Spread peanut butter on banana slices.

Nutritional Value:

Calories: 200

Protein: 4g

Carbohydrates: 30g

Fat: 8g

Fiber: 4g

Cooking Time: 5 minutes

9. Mixed Nuts and Dried Fruit

Ingredients:

1/4 cup mixed nuts (unsalted)

1/4 cup dried fruit (such as raisins, cranberries, or apricots)

Preparation:

1. Combine mixed nuts and dried fruit in a bowl.

Nutritional Value:

Calories: 220

Protein: 5g

Carbohydrates: 28g

Fat: 12g

Fiber: 4g

Cooking Time: 2 minutes

10. Chia Pudding

Ingredients:

1/4 cup chia seeds

1 cup almond milk (unsweetened)

1 tablespoon honey

1/2 teaspoon vanilla extract

Preparation:

1. In a bowl, mix chia seeds, almond milk, honey, and vanilla extract.

2. Stir well and refrigerate for at least 4 hours, or overnight, until it thickens.

Nutritional Value:

Calories: 200

Protein: 4g

Carbohydrates: 28g

Fat: 8g

Fiber: 10g

Cooking Time: 10 minutes (plus chilling time)

Desserts:

1. Berry Yogurt Parfait

Ingredients:

1 cup plain Greek yogurt

1/2 cup mixed berries (strawberries, blueberries, raspberries)

1 tablespoon honey

2 tablespoons granola (optional)

Preparation:

1. In a glass or bowl, layer Greek yogurt, mixed berries, and honey.

2. Repeat layers as desired.

3. Top with granola if using.

Nutritional Value:

Calories: 200

Protein: 15g

Carbohydrates: 30g

Fat: 3g

Fiber: 5g

Preparation Time: 5 minutes

2. Baked Apples with Cinnamon

Ingredients:

4 apples, cored

1/4 cup raisins

1 teaspoon cinnamon

1 tablespoon honey

1/4 cup chopped nuts (optional)

Preparation:

1. Preheat oven to 375°F (190°C).

2. Place apples in a baking dish.

3. Mix raisins, cinnamon, and honey in a bowl.

4. Stuff each apple with raisin mixture.

5. Bake for 25-30 minutes, until apples are tender.

6. Sprinkle with chopped nuts if desired.

Nutritional Value:

Calories: 180

Protein: 2g

Carbohydrates: 40g

Fat: 3g

Fiber: 6g

Cooking Time: 30 minutes

3. Dark Chocolate-Dipped Strawberries

Ingredients:

12 strawberries, washed and dried

2 oz dark chocolate (70% cocoa or higher)

Preparation:

1. Line a baking sheet with parchment paper.

2. Melt dark chocolate in a microwave-safe bowl in 30-second intervals, stirring until smooth.

3. Dip each strawberry into melted chocolate, coating halfway.

4. Place on parchment paper and let cool until chocolate hardens.

Nutritional Value:

Calories: 150

Protein: 2g

Carbohydrates: 20g

Fat: 8g

Fiber: 4g

Preparation Time: 15 minutes

4. Banana Ice Cream

Ingredients:

2 ripe bananas, peeled and sliced

1/4 cup almond milk (unsweetened)

1 teaspoon vanilla extract

Toppings: chopped nuts, berries (optional)

Preparation:

1. Freeze banana slices until firm, about 2 hours.

2. In a blender or food processor, blend frozen banana slices, almond milk, and vanilla extract until smooth.

3. Serve immediately topped with chopped nuts or berries if desired.

Nutritional Value:

Calories: 180

Protein: 3g

Carbohydrates: 40g

Fat: 2g

Fiber: 5g

Preparation Time: 5 minutes (plus freezing time)

5. Chia Seed Pudding with Berries

Ingredients:

1/4 cup chia seeds

1 cup almond milk (unsweetened)

1 tablespoon honey

1/2 teaspoon vanilla extract

1/2 cup mixed berries (strawberries, blueberries, raspberries)

Preparation:

1. In a bowl, mix chia seeds, almond milk, honey, and vanilla extract.

2. Stir well and refrigerate for at least 4 hours, or overnight, until it thickens.

3. Serve topped with mixed berries.

Nutritional Value:

Calories: 220

Protein: 6g

Carbohydrates: 30g

Fat: 10g

Fiber: 10g

Preparation Time: 5 minutes (plus chilling time)

6. Grilled Pineapple with Cinnamon

Ingredients:

1 pineapple, peeled and cored

1 teaspoon cinnamon

1 tablespoon honey

Preparation:

1. Preheat grill to medium-high heat.

2. Cut pineapple into rings.

3. Grill pineapple rings for 2-3 minutes on each side, until grill marks appear.

4. Sprinkle with cinnamon and drizzle with honey before serving.

Nutritional Value:

Calories: 150

Protein: 1g

Carbohydrates: 40g

Fat: 0g

Fiber: 3g

Cooking Time: 10 minutes

7. Mango Sorbet

Ingredients:

2 ripe mangoes, peeled and diced

1/4 cup water

1 tablespoon honey

Juice of 1 lime

Preparation:

1. Place diced mangoes in a blender.

2. Add water, honey, and lime juice.

3. Blend until smooth.

4. Pour into a shallow dish and freeze for 2-3 hours, stirring occasionally, until firm.

Nutritional Value:

Calories: 120

Protein: 1g

Carbohydrates: 30g

Fat: 0g

Fiber: 3g

Preparation Time: 10 minutes (plus freezing time)

8. Berry Frozen Yogurt Bites

Ingredients:

1 cup plain Greek yogurt

1/2 cup mixed berries (strawberries, blueberries, raspberries)

1 tablespoon honey

Preparation:

1. Line a mini muffin tin with paper liners.

2. In a bowl, mix Greek yogurt, mixed berries, and honey.

3. Spoon yogurt mixture into muffin tin compartments.

4. Freeze for 2-3 hours, until firm.

Nutritional Value:

Calories: 100

Protein: 5g

Carbohydrates: 15g

Fat: 2g

Fiber: 2g

Preparation Time: 10 minutes (plus freezing time)

9. Lemon Poppy Seed Muffins

Ingredients:

1 cup whole wheat flour

1/2 cup almond flour

1/4 cup honey

1/4 cup plain Greek yogurt

1/4 cup almond milk (unsweetened)

2 tablespoons olive oil

1 egg

Zest of 1 lemon

Juice of 1 lemon

1 tablespoon poppy seeds

1 teaspoon baking powder

1/2 teaspoon baking soda

Pinch of salt

Preparation:

1. Preheat oven to 350°F (175°C). Line a muffin tin with paper liners.

2. In a bowl, whisk together honey, Greek yogurt, almond milk, olive oil, egg, lemon zest, and lemon juice.

3. In another bowl, combine whole wheat flour, almond flour, poppy seeds, baking powder, baking soda, and salt.

4. Gradually add dry ingredients to wet ingredients, stirring until just combined.

5. Spoon batter into muffin tin compartments.

6. Bake for 18-20 minutes, until a toothpick inserted into the center comes out clean.

Nutritional Value:

Calories: 150

Protein: 5g

Carbohydrates: 20g

Fat: 6g

Fiber: 3g

Cooking Time: 30 minutes

10. Oatmeal Raisin Cookies

Ingredients:

1 cup rolled oats

1/2 cup whole wheat flour

1/2 cup raisins

1/4 cup honey

1/4 cup unsweetened applesauce

1/4 cup olive oil

1 egg

1 teaspoon vanilla extract

1/2 teaspoon cinnamon

1/2 teaspoon baking soda

Pinch of salt

Preparation:

1. Preheat oven to 350°F (175°C). Line a baking sheet with parchment paper.

2. In a bowl, combine rolled oats, whole wheat flour, raisins, honey, applesauce, olive oil, egg, vanilla extract, cinnamon, baking soda, and salt.

3. Drop spoonfuls of dough onto the baking sheet.

4. Flatten each cookie slightly with a fork.

5. Bake for 10-12 minutes, until edges are golden brown.

Nutritional Value:

Calories: 140

Protein: 3g

Carbohydrates: 20g

Fat: 6g

Fiber: 2g

Cooking Time: 20 minutes

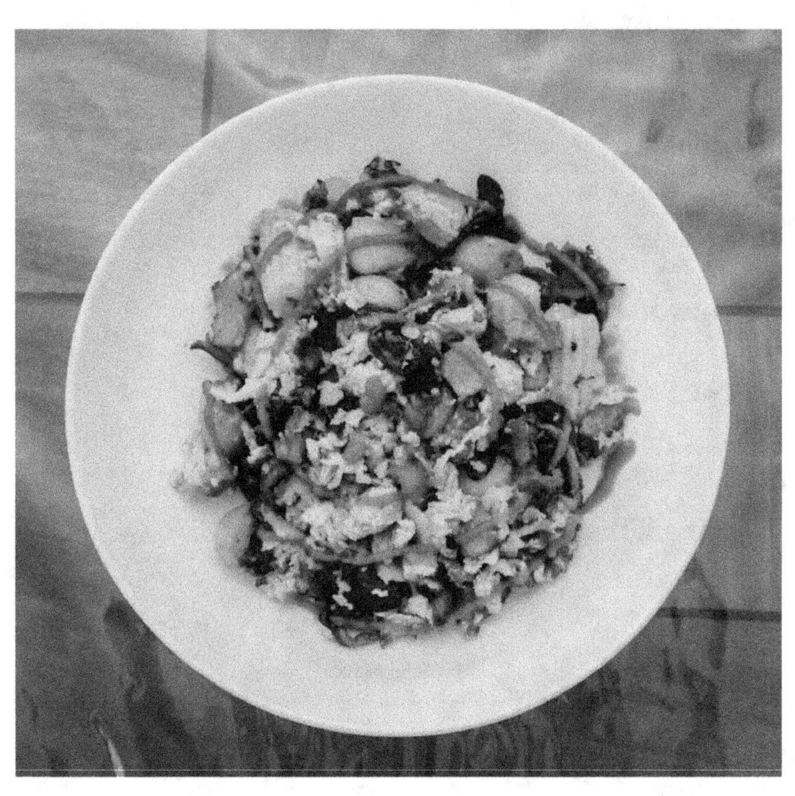

CONCLUSION

In embracing the DASH (Dietary Approaches to Stop Hypertension) diet, you embark on a journey towards not just better health, but a revitalized lifestyle that prioritizes well-being. Throughout this cookbook, we've explored a plethora of nutritious and flavorful recipes designed to lower blood pressure, reduce inflammation, and support overall heart health.

The foundation of the DASH diet lies in its emphasis on whole foods rich in nutrients, such as fruits, vegetables, lean proteins, and whole grains, while limiting sodium, refined sugars, and saturated fats. Each recipe here has been crafted to not only meet these dietary guidelines but also to tantalize your taste buds and make healthy eating a joy, not a chore.

By adopting the DASH diet, you not only reduce your risk of hypertension and cardiovascular diseases but also promote weight management and improve overall vitality. Scientifically endorsed, this diet has been proven effective in numerous studies, offering benefits beyond just heart health—it supports brain function, bone health, and reduces the risk of certain cancers.

As you embark on this culinary journey, remember that every meal is an opportunity to nourish your body and soul. Whether you're starting fresh or looking to enhance your existing healthy habits, the DASH diet provides a sustainable path towards longevity and vitality.

So, take charge of your health today. Let this cookbook be your guide to a delicious and healthful lifestyle. Embrace the DASH diet not just as a diet, but as a life-affirming choice that empowers you to live your best life, every day.

Special Motivation

Embrace the DASH diet as your ally in health, and witness the transformative power of food. Every bite you take brings you closer to a healthier future—where vitality, joy, and longevity await. Start today and reap the rewards for years to come.

Medical View

From a medical perspective, adopting the DASH diet offers a significant advantage in managing hypertension and reducing cardiovascular risk factors. Its balanced approach ensures you receive essential nutrients while maintaining healthy blood pressure levels. By making this diet a part of your life, you invest in a future of robust health and well-being

Weekly Planner

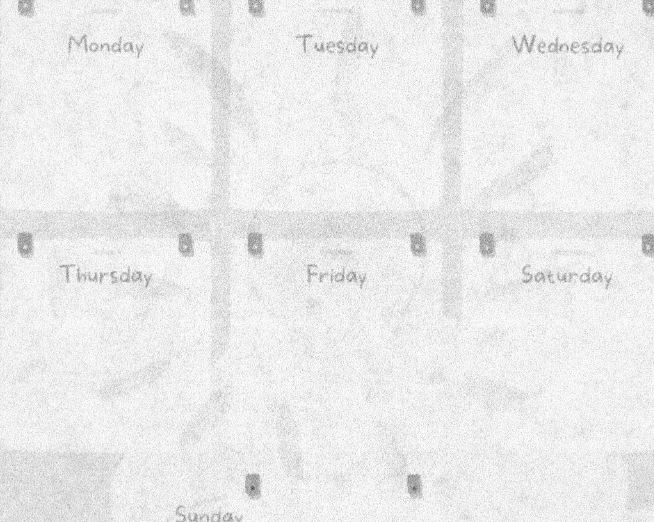

Weekly Planner

Monday

Tuesday

Wednesday

Thursday

Friday

Saturday

Sunday

Weekly Planner

Monday

Tuesday

Wednesday

Thursday

Friday

Saturday

Sunday

Weekly Planner

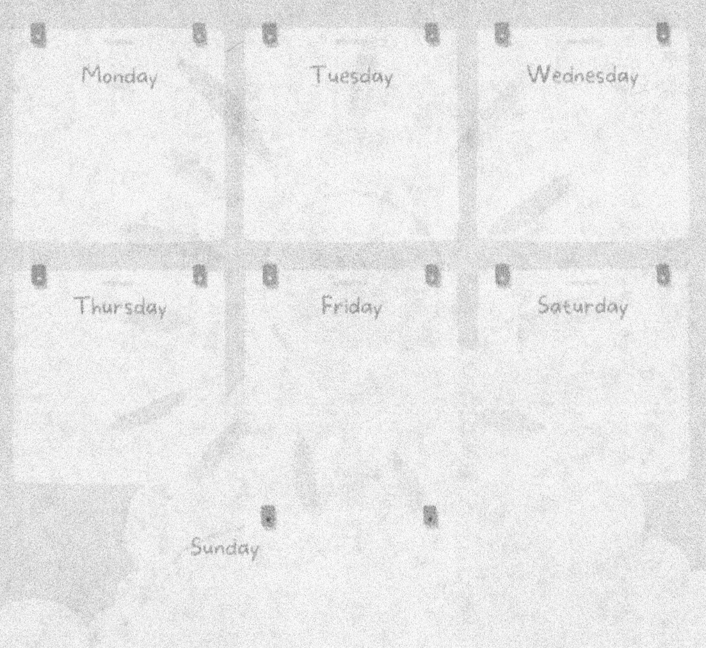

Weekly Planner

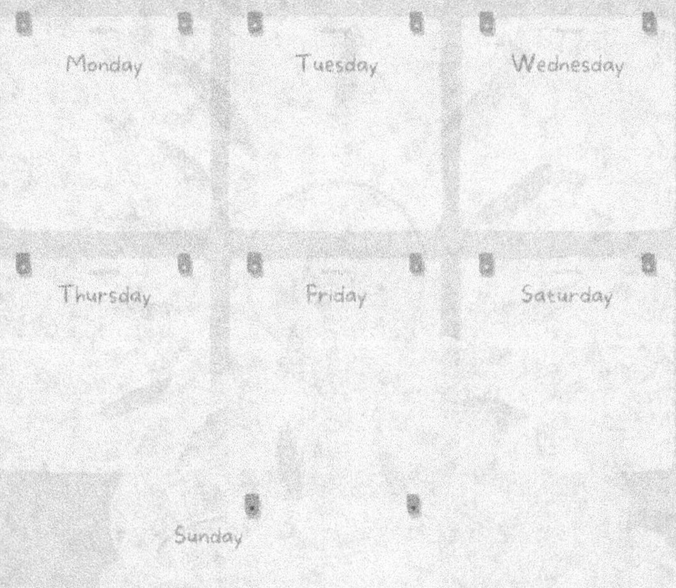

Weekly Planner

Monday

Tuesday

Wednesday

Thursday

Friday

Saturday

Sunday

Weekly Planner

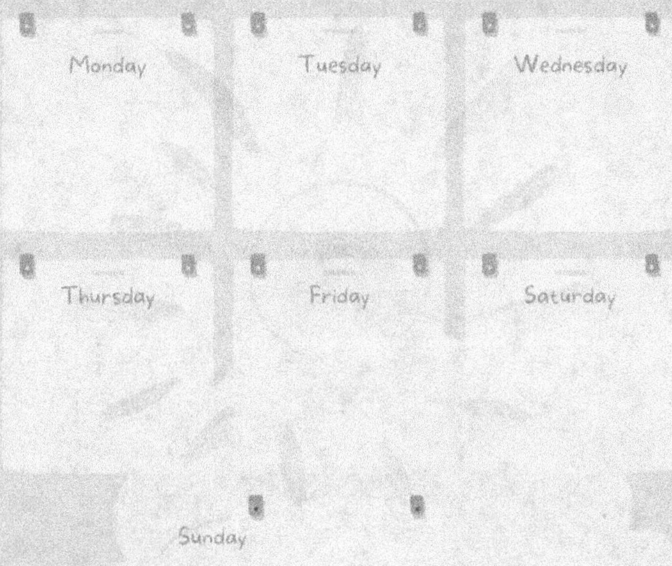

Weekly Planner

Monday

Tuesday

Wednesday

Thursday

Friday

Saturday

Sunday

Weekly Planner

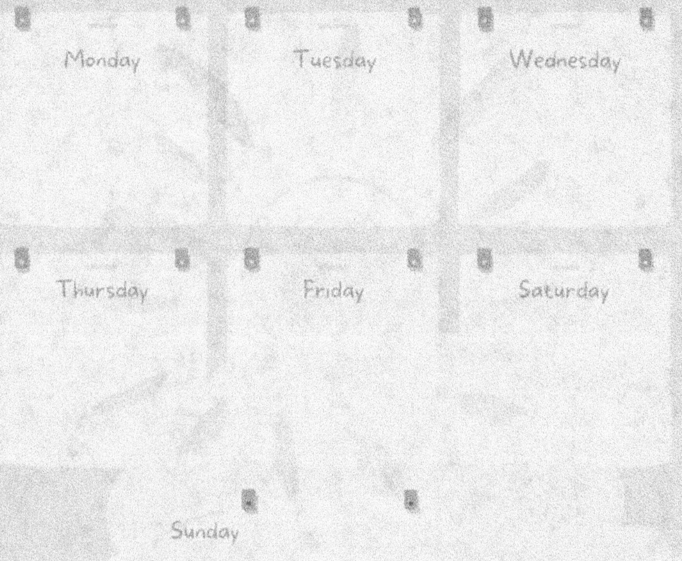

Weekly Planner

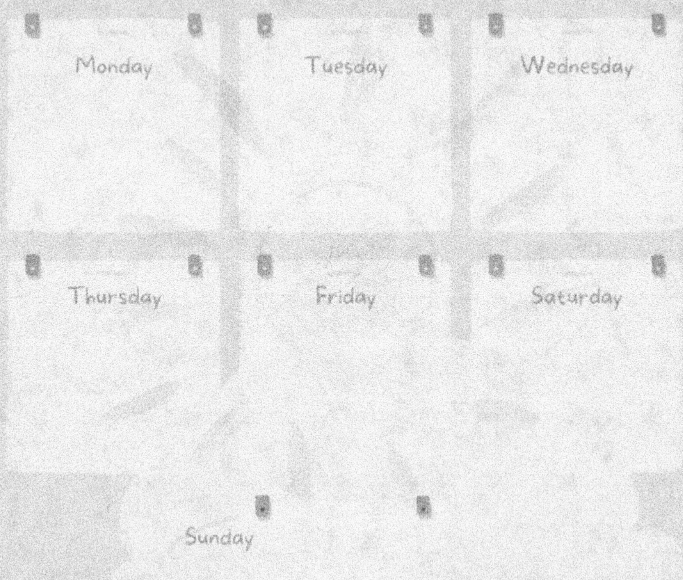

Weekly Planner

Monday

Tuesday

Wednesday

Thursday

Friday

Saturday

Sunday

Weekly Planner

Monday

Tuesday

Wednesday

Thursday

Friday

Saturday

Sunday

Weekly
Planner

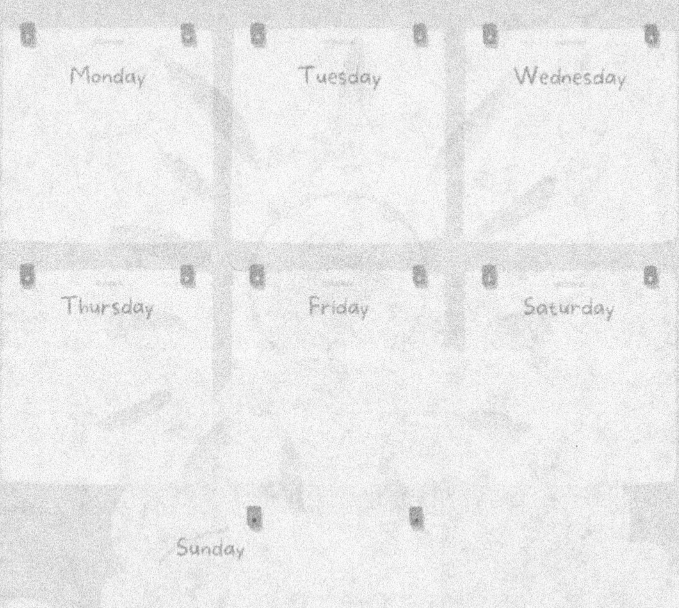

Weekly Planner

Monday

Tuesday

Wednesday

Thursday

Friday

Saturday

Sunday

www.ingramcontent.com/pod-product-compliance
Lightning Source LLC
Chambersburg PA
CBHW050805250726

48653CB00006B/2087